# YOUR KNOWLEDGE HAS VALUE

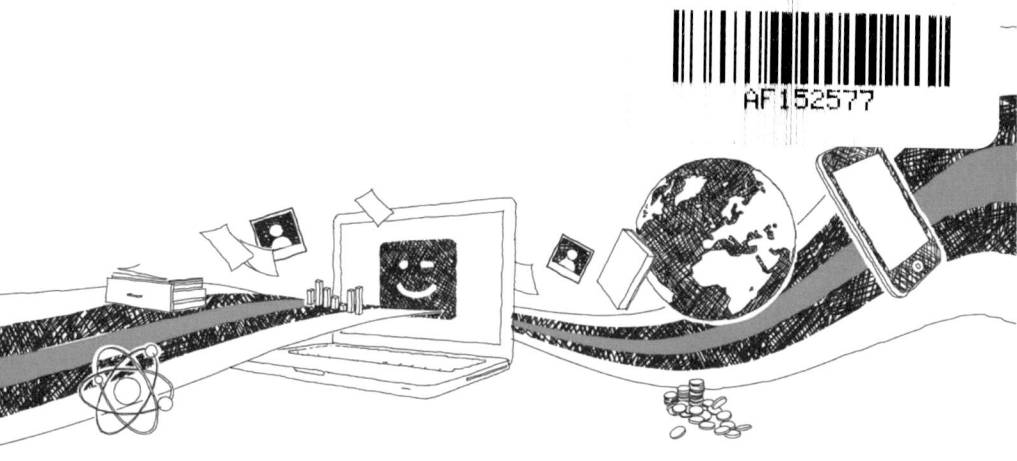
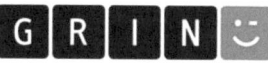

# Sustainability in e-Health. Overview and emerging challenges

Jan Harder

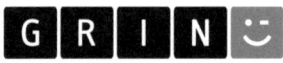

**Bibliographic information published by the German National Library:**

The German National Library lists this publication in the National Bibliography; detailed bibliographic data are available on the Internet at http://dnb.dnb.de.

ISBN: 9783346560575
This book is also available as an ebook.

Print and binding: Books on Demand GmbH, Norderstedt, Germany
Printed on acid-free paper from responsible sources.

The present work has been carefully prepared. Nevertheless, authors and publishers do not incur liability for the correctness of information, notes, links and advice as well as any printing errors.

GRIN web shop: https://www.grin.com/document/1160779

# Sustainability in e-Health: Overview and emerging challenges

## Individual Assignment INFN25 Autumn 2021

Author: Jan Harder

## Abstract

Doctor visits and hospital stays are often characterized by inefficient processes, for patients and doctors as well as for hospitals and insurance companies. Enabled by new technologies, many of these processes can be digitized and thus made more efficient, accurate, and sustainable. The purpose of this article is to provide an overview of how e-health services can contribute to greater sustainability through information and communications technology, both for the environment and for society, as well to identify areas where e-health applications can still be optimized or where new problems arise.

# Table of Contents

# 1 Introduction

Digitization in healthcare continues to permeate all areas. For a long time now, it has not just been about pure telemetry, i.e. electronic communication between the involved parties, but also innovative systems such as the use of machine learning to detect irregularities in X-ray images (Kassania et al., 2021). This is also reflected in the increasing interest of companies and investors in the field of e-health. The amount of annual global investment in the digital health industry has increased from one billion US dollars in 2010 to 21.6 billion in 2020 (StartUp Health, 2021). This was also driven by the huge increase of 55% from 2019 to 2020, due to a very strong interest in e-health solutions during the COVID-19 pandemic (StartUp Health, 2021).

E-health solutions offer many advantages for patients, doctors, health insurers, and hospitals. Processes become more efficient through digital communication, patients can receive remote diagnoses via video chat and have digital patient records, and doctors are supported in diagnoses and freed from bureaucratic tasks and can devote more time to their patients. However, due to the continued importance of the healthcare system to society and its long-term planning, consideration must also be given to how e-health can be made as sustainable as possible.

# 2 E-Health

The term e-health describes a very broad set of technologies for digitizing the medical sector. A very common definition of e-health, judging by the citations, is the one given by Eysenbach (2001, p. 1): *"e-health is an emerging field in the intersection of medical informatics, public health and business, referring to health services and information delivered or enhanced through the Internet and related technologies"*, such as enhancing quality, education or ethics, to show that e-health also describes the mission of using it to create improvements in health care (Eysenbach, 2001). Shaw et al. (2007) also identified three domains of e-health in their interviews with health industry professionals. *Health in Our Hands* describes the use of mobile devices for obtaining information on the one hand and wearables for measuring medical data on the other. *Interacting for Health* refers to communication through information and communication technology (ICT), such as video consultations or interactive online learning platforms for medical staff. *Data Enabling Health* includes the generation, storage, processing, and use of medical data. When data is incorporated into decision-making, the quality and precision of medical interventions can be increased and human error minimized (Shaw et al., 2007). Another term that often comes up in the same context is m-health, which limits e-health to the use of mobile technology (Free et al., 2010).

The definitions show that the term e-health is very broadly defined, since the digitization of all medical processes is at its core, but overlaps primarily in the areas of digital communication and information procurement. In the following, the numerous use cases of e-health and their advantages will be highlighted, but also the risks that arise.

## 2.1 Opportunities and Challenges

Because e-health is such a broad term, the benefits also extend to many areas and actors in the healthcare system. Enabled by ICT, patients can be monitored from home. Pare et al. (2007) state that reliable data is collected for more patients and more patients seek medical help when they can stay at home. This and video telephony with medical staff not only saves patients time but also reduces the number of hospital or doctor visits, which in turn can save costs (Schweizer & Synowiec, 2012; Stroetmann, 2017). Catewell and Sheikh (2009) concluded in their study that providing health portals where patients can view their own health data and have easy access to reliable medical information will increase their health awareness and give them and their physicians faster access to their data. Another advantage of mobile e-health devices is that information can be personalized and given on demand. For example, while a doctor can recommend what to do in the event of a high pulse, a smartwatch with a heart rate monitor can give the appropriate information when the case arises (Van Gemert-Pijnen et al., 2018). In addition, technology is easy to scale compared to medical personnel, which would be especially beneficial for large or unpredictable campaigns (Van Gemert-Pijnen et al., 2018).

Nevertheless, the use of e-health also carries risks, as patients' health and personal data are directly affected. Because e-health has been promoted and developed so rapidly, errors can also occur in e-health applications or errors can arise due to incorrect use by healthcare professionals (Han et al., 2015; Catwell & Sheikh, 2009). Therefore, good usability is needed, because otherwise, not only will errors occur that can hurt patients, but the application will also take longer, or professionals will not accept and use the application (Sousa & Dunn Lopez, 2017). In addition, the hardware and Internet connection must be fast enough to not slow down the efficiency of the applications (Ambrose, Braithwaite & Wilson, 2011). Since sensitive data is involved, particular emphasis must be placed on privacy and IT security. This is also shown by recent cybercrime cases in which sensitive data was stolen and millions of dollars in damage were caused by forged prescriptions (Brewin, 2009). To minimize these risks, Ossebaard et al. (2013) issued recommendations for action for developers and responsible parties, recommending that all stakeholders be made aware of the risks and research them further, as well as creating portals for reporting errors and using risk management tools.

## 2.2 Required ICT Components

In order to develop such complex and highly interconnected e-health systems, a number of technologies need to be integrated. In addition to the procurement of hardware, special software must also be set up for the healthcare sector. Since an average clinical center already has to process and store large amounts of data, for example through X-ray images, which are enriched by machine learning processes, appropriate databases must be made available (Amato et al., 2019). Also enabled by machine learning, more precisely natural language processing, chatbots can be programmed to provide patients with answers to frequently asked questions around the clock (Amato et al., 2019). To guarantee data security, such as protection against data theft, availability, or integrity, blockchain solutions can be used, which with the help of smart contracts can ensure that only patients can view or release their data, without third parties having to process or store data (Rifi et al., 2017). This includes using ICT systems to determine which employees have access to which data. In order to be able to manage all data, processes, and authorizations, a central platform should be used in which data can also be imported from wearables, sensors or external databases or messages can be sent to other m-health devices (Alberts et al., 2014). Since healthcare facilities do not always have sufficiently powerful data centers, software as a service, platform as a service, and infrastructure as a service solutions can be used for this purpose (Alberts et al., 2014).

# 3 Sustainable E-Health

Sustainability has many different definitions in the literature, but many express the same as the definition of the World Commission on Environment and Development (1987, p. 39): "*Sustainable development seeks to meet the needs and aspirations of the present without compromising the ability to meet those of the future*".

Looking at the three dimensions of sustainability, social, economic, and environmental (Kuhlman & Farrington, 2010), it quickly becomes clear that sustainability is inextricably linked to healthcare and ICT. Although sustainability is difficult to measure and the different dimensions are difficult to balance against each other, an overview can be given of how e-health affects sustainability.

Malmodin and Lundén (2018) calculated in their study with data from 2015 that the ICT sector is responsible for 1.4% of global $CO_2$ emissions and 3.6% of global energy consumption, observing that the production and use of ICT devices are steadily increasing. This has a negative impact not only on the climate and wildlife but also on society, especially on developing countries, which are more affected by climate change even though they produce less greenhouse gases (Patz et al., 2007). However, a focus on the social and environmental dimensions without looking at the profitability of e-health companies would not be beneficial either, as companies need to remain profitable to positively impact society and the climate in the long run (Giovanni & Zabietti, 2013). The link between e-health and sustainability is also reflected in the United Nations Sustainable Development Goals (2007), in particular in the "Good Health and Well-Being", "Gender Equality", "Industry, Innovation and Infrastructure", and "Climate Action" goals.

ICT is seen both as a cause of problems in the context of sustainability and as an enabler for innovation and the possibility of designing processes and products more sustainably. In the following, an overview will be given of how ICT already promotes sustainability in the healthcare sector and how e-health innovation can be used to promote sustainability even further.

## 3.1 How E-Health contributes to Sustainability

The positive impact of switching to e-health solutions on the environment is already visible. A study by Yellowless et al. (2010) showed that 13,000 video calls made saved 7.6 million kilometers of travel and 1,700 tons of $CO_2$ emissions. Holmner et al. (2014) also conclude that the use of e-health, in the form of videotelephony, is worthwhile even for short journeys if it means that the car is no longer needed. However, they also note that $CO_2$ emissions depend heavily on which means of transport is replaced, how long the video calls last, and what bandwidth is used. In addition, the digitalization of healthcare processes, such as digital files or digital communication between doctors, hospitals, and patients, saves large amounts of paper, thus slowing down deforestation, which contributes significantly to climate change (Holmner et al., 2012).

The society also benefits from the use of e-health, through improved medical care and increased quality of life, for example through shorter hospital stays or the ability to be monitored by sensors in the event of illness at home (Fanta, Pretorius & Erasmus, 2015). In addition, the risk of

4

communicable diseases is reduced if fewer consultations take place on-site. In part, e-health also contributes to equity. People living in rural areas with long distances to health centers have easier access to health services (Fanta, Pretorius & Erasmus, 2015). Especially in developing countries where medical staff and resources are limited, increased efficiency, e-learning platforms, and telemedicine can benefit. Through online appointment scheduling, discrimination can also be limited as appointments are automatically assigned. In addition, through e-health, health information is available online to everyone, which can reduce educational disparities.

As explained earlier, the introduction of e-health has already resulted in cost savings in some cases. However, due to the complexities of healthcare cost coverage structures, cost analyses are often very complicated and in some cases not yet possible (Sanyal et al., 2018). To bring innovation to the healthcare market, startups play a major role, as they are often able to develop disruptive technologies much faster than established companies (Schaltegger & Wagner, 2011; Garbuio & Lin, 2019). Although startups are held back by strict approval procedures in the healthcare system and the complicated cost coverage structure by health insurers (Rinsche, 2017), startups can also take advantage of this because it is easier to convince users of e-health apps if their health insurer covers the costs, as is the case in Germany, for example (Hawkins, 2020).

## 3.2 How to make E-Health more sustainable

Although e-health is already contributing to sustainability in many areas, there are still many areas where challenges remain. There is no shortage of sustainable e-health technologies and innovations, but implementation is hindered by strict regulations, lack of IT infrastructure or sufficient technical education, ethical concerns, and financing issues.

Sustainability can be enhanced even further by incorporating the principles of Green IT. Green IT describes the conscious consideration of sustainable aspects in IT products, which not only protects the environment but also saves costs through lower power consumption (Murugesan, 2008). Dash et al. (2019) estimate that by 2020, 40,000 billion terabytes of data will be stored worldwide by the healthcare system. Since storing and processing such large amounts of data is extremely energy-intensive, green cloud computing principles, such as virtualization of data centers, should be applied (Baliga, 2011). To make sustainable decisions, monitoring software should be used that is designed to measure environmentally relevant values (Malmodin & Lundén, 2018).

Social aspects must also be taken into account to a greater extent in the development of e-health applications, for example through ethics committees. For example, AI-driven systems often exhibit biases against certain genders or races because the AI models have been trained with biased data (Parikh, Teeple & Navathe, 2019). There is also a need to ensure that everyone can use e-health applications, as people with lower incomes, low education, disabilities, or the elderly often cannot easily navigate IT applications (Viswanath & Kreuter, 2007; Eng, 2002). To change this, offerings need to be provided in simple language and assistance must be ensured. For developing countries to benefit from e-health, they must be provided with financial support and IT specialists.

Start-ups in the e-health sector are struggling with the strict regulations in the health care sector and the cost coverage by health care providers (Rinsche, 2017). Reiher, Oemig, and Dahlweid (2008) therefore suggest that research into the cost-benefit ratio of e-health application needs to be explored more by researchers to convince healthcare providers to invest in the start-ups. For start-ups to take advantage of their disruptive innovations despite strong regulations, Herrmann et al. (2018) suggest teaming up with other companies to keep up with the experience of established companies.

# 4 Conclusion

This study has shown that e-health applications not only promise higher quality in medicine but have already been proven to contribute to the achievement of sustainability goals. In the environmental, social, and economic dimensions, e-health offers promising solutions. However, at the same time, the literature suggests that the potential of sustainable e-health is not yet exhausted and that new problems may arise from the introduction of e-health, such as biases in AI applications. Future research should continue to explore frameworks and monitoring software to provide data and recommendations for action in the development and operation of e-health applications to facilitate sustainable decision-making. In addition, the economic benefits of e-health solutions need to be further explored to convince healthcare providers to invest in them and to further optimize costs.

# References

Alberts, R., Fogwill, T., Botra, A., & Cretty, M. (2014). An integrative ICT platform for eHealth. *2014 IST-Africa Conference Proceedings*, pp. 1-8, Availabe Online: https://ieeexplore.ieee.org/abstract/document/6880650/ [Accessed: October 22, 2021]

Amato, F., Marrone, S., Moscato, V., Piantadosi, G., Picariello, A., & Sansone, C. (2019). HOLMeS: eHealth in the Big Data and Deep Learning Era, *Information*, vol. 10, no. 2, pp. 1-13, Availabe Online: https://doi.org/10.3390/info10020034 [Accessed: October 22, 2021]

Ambrose, H., Braithwaite, M., & Wilson, J. (2011). Perceived benefits of ehealth implementations to healthcare workers and patients, *Telecommunications Journal of Australia*, vol. 61, p.4, Available Online: https://researchbank.swinburne.edu.au/file/753fe8e0-8367-4c6c-a926-bb4b1f8d4004/1/tja_2011_vol61_no3_43-ambrose_etal.pdf [Accessed: October 21, 2021]

Baliga, J., Ayre, R. W. A., Hinton, K., & Tucker, R. S. (2011). Green Cloud Computing: Balancing Energy in Processing, Storage, and Transport, *Proceedings of the IEEE*, vol. 99, no. 1, pp. 149-167, Available Online: https://ieeexplore.ieee.org/abstract/document/5559320 [Accessed: October 25, 2021]

Brewin, B. (2009). Cyber criminals overseas steal US electronic health records, Nextgov, Availabe Online: https://www.nextgov.com/cio-briefing/2008/05/cyber-criminals-overseas-steal-us-electronic-health-records/42081/ [Accessed: October 22, 2021]

Catwell, L., & Sheikh, A. (2009). Evaluating eHealth Interventions: The Need for Continuous Systemic Evaluation, *PLOS Medicine*, vol. 6, no. 8, p. 2, Available Online: https://doi.org/10.1371/journal.pmed.1000126 [Accessed: October 21, 2021]

Dash, S., Shakyawar, S.K., Sharma, & Kaushik, S. (2019). Big data in healthcare: management, analysis and future prospects, *J Big Data*, vol. 6, no. 54, Available Online: https://doi.org/10.1186/s40537-019-0217-0 [Accessed: October 25, 2021]

Eng, T. R. (2002). eHealth research and evaluation: challenges and opportunities, *Journal of health communication*, vol. 7, no. 4, pp. 267-272, Available Online: https://www.tandfonline.com/doi/pdf/10.1080/10810730290001747 [Accessed: October 21, 2021]

Eysenbach, G. (2001). What is e-health?, *J Med Internet Res*, vol. 3, no. 2, p.1, Available Online: https://www.jmir.org/2001/2/e20 [Accessed: October 20, 2021]

Fanta, G., Pretorius, L., & Erasmus, L. (2015). An evaluation of ehealth systems implementation frameworks for sustainability in resource constrained environments: A literature review, *International Association for Management of Technology (IAMOT)*, pp. 1046-1063, Available Online: https://www.academia.edu/download/46611485/AN_EVALUATION_OF_EHEALTH_SYSTEMS_IMPLEME20160619-7479-1whkdut.pdf [Accessed: October 23, 2021]

Filchev, R., Pavlova, D., Dimova, R., & Dovramadjiev, T. (2022). Healthcare System Sustainability by Application of Advanced Technologies in Telemedicine and eHealth, *Human Interaction, Emerging Technologies and Future Systems V. Lecture Notes in Networks and Systems*, vol 319, pp. 1027-1033, Available Online: https://doi.org/10.1007/978-3-030-85540-6_129 [Accessed: October 23, 2021]

Free, C., Phillips, G., Felix, L., Galli, L., Patel, V., & Edwards, P. (2010). The effectiveness of M-health technologies for improving health and health services: a systematic review protocol, *BMC Res Notes*, vol. 3, no. 250, Available Online: https://doi.org/10.1186/1756-0500-3-250 [Accessed: October 20, 2021]

Garbuio, M., Lin, N. (2019). Artificial Intelligence as a Growth Engine for Health Care Startups: Emerging Business Models, *California Management Review*, vo. 61, no. 2, pp. 59-83, Available Online: https://journals.sagepub.com/doi/full/10.1177/0008125618811931 [Accessed: October 24, 2021]

Gatzoulis, L., & Iakovidis, I. (2007). Wearable and Portable eHealth Systems, *IEEE Engineering in Medicine and Biology Magazine*, vol. 26, no. 5, pp. 51-56, Available Online: https://ieeexplore.ieee.org/abstract/document/4312668 [Accessed: October 22, 2021]

Gibson, R. B. (2001). Specification of sustainability-based environmental assessment decision criteria and implications for determining" significance" in environmental assessment, p. 10, Available Online: https://static.twoday.net/NE1BOKU0607/files/Gibson_Sustainability-EA.pdf [Accessed: October 23, 2021]

Giovannoni E., & Fabietti G. (2013). What Is Sustainability? A Review of the Concept and Its Applications, *Integrated Reporting*, pp. 21-40. Available Online https://doi.org/10.1007/978-3-319-02168-3_2 [Accessed: October 20, 2021]

Han, Y. Y., Carcillo, J. A., Venkataraman, S. T., Clark, R. S., Watson, R. S., Nguyen, T. C., Bayir, H., & Orr, R, A. (2015). Unexpected increased mortality after implementation of a commercially sold computerized physician order entry system, *Pediatrics*, vol 112, no. 6, pp. 1506-1512, Available Online: https://pubmed.ncbi.nlm.nih.gov/16322178/ [Accessed: October 21, 2021]

Hawkins, L. (2020). Health apps now available on prescription in Germany, Available Online: https://healthcareglobal.com/digital-healthcare/health-apps-now-available-prescription-germany [Accessed: October 24, 2021]

Herrmann, M., Boehme, P., Mondritzki, T., Ehlers, J.P., Kavadias, S., & Truebel H. (2018). Digital transformation and disruption of the health care sector: Internet-based observational study, *Journal of Medical Internet Research*, vol. 20, no. 3, Available Online: https://www.jmir.org/2018/3/e104/ [Accessed: October 25, 2021]

Holmner, Å., Ebi, K.L., Lazuardi, L., & Nilsson, M. (2014). Carbon Footprint of Telemedicine Solutions - Unexplored Opportunity for Reducing Carbon Emissions in the Health Sector, *PLOS ONE*, vol. 9, no. 9, pp.6-9, Available Online: https://doi.org/10.1371/journal.pone.0105040 [Accessed: October 24, 2021]

Holmner, Å., Rocklöv, J., Ng, N., & Nilsson, M. (2012) Climate change and eHealth: a promising strategy for health sector mitigation and adaptation, *Global Health Action*, vol. 5, no. 1, pp. 1-6, Available Online: https://www.tandfonline.com/doi/full/10.3402/gha.v5i0.18428 [Accessed: October 24, 2021]

Kassania, S. H., Kassanib, P. H., Wesolowskic, M. J., Schneidera, K. A., & Detersa, R. (2021). Automatic Detection of Coronavirus Disease (COVID-19) in X-ray and CT Images: A Machine Learning Based Approach, *Biocybernetics and Biomedical Engineering*, vol. 41, no. 3, pp. 867-879, Available Online: https://doi.org/10.1016/j.bbe.2021.05.013 [Accessed: October 25, 2021]

Khoja, S., Durrani, H., Nayani, P., & Fahim, A. (2012). Scope of Policy Issues in eHealth: Results From a Structured Literature Review, *J Med Internet Res*, vol. 14, no. 1, Available Online: https://www.jmir.org/2012/1/e34 [Accessed: October 24, 2021]

Kuhlman, T., & Farrington J. (2010). What is Sustainability?, *Sustainability*, vol. 2, no. 11, pp. 3436-3448, Available Online: https://www.mdpi.com/2071-1050/2/11/3436 [Accessed: October 23, 2021]

Malmodin, J., & Lundén, D. (2018). The Energy and Carbon Footprint of the Global ICT and E&M Sectors 2010–2015, *Sustainability*, vol. 10, no. 9, p. 28, Available Online: https://doi.org/10.3390/su10093027 [Accessed: October 23, 2021]

Murugesan, S. (2008). Harnessing Green IT: Principles and Practices, *IT Professional*, vol. 10, no. 1, pp. 24-33, Available Online: https://ieeexplore.ieee.org/abstract/document/4446673 [Accessed: October 25, 2021]

Ossebaard, H. C., De Bruijn, A. C. P., Van Gemert-Pijnen, J. E., & Geertsma, R. E. (2013). Risks related to the use of eHealth technologies: An exploratory study, National Institute for Public Health and the Environment of the Netherlands, p. 53, Availabe Online: https://rivm.openrepository.com/handle/10029/305616 [Accessed: October 21, 2021]

Pagliari, C., Sloan, D., Gregor, P., Sullivan, F., Detmer, D., Kahan, J., Oortwijn, W., & MacGillivray, S. (2005). What Is eHealth (4): A Scoping Exercise to Map the Field, *J Med Internet Res*, vol. 7, no. 1, p. 1, Availabe Online: https://www.jmir.org/2005/1/e9 [Accessed: October 22, 2021]

Paré, G., Jaana, M., & Sicotte, C. (2007). Systematic Review of Home Telemonitoring for Chronic Diseases: The Evidence Base, *Journal of the American Medical Informatics Association*, vol. 14, no. 3, pp. 269–277. Available Online: https://doi.org/10.1197/jamia.M2270 [Accessed: October 21, 2021]

Parikh, R. B., Teeple, S., & Navathe, A. S. (2019). Addressing Bias in Artificial Intelligence in Health Care, *JAMA*, vol. 322, no. 24, pp. 2377–2378, Available Online: https://jamanetwork.com/journals/jama/article-abstract/2756196 [Accessed: October 25, 2021]

Patz, J.A., Gibbs, H.K., Foley, J.A., Rogers, J. V., & Smith, K.R. (2007). Climate Change and Global Health: Quantifying a Growing Ethical Crisis, *EcoHealth*, vol. 4, pp. 397–405, Available Online: https://doi.org/10.1007/s10393-007-0141-1 [Accessed: October 23, 2021]

Reiher, M., Oemig, F., & Dahlweid, M. F. (2008). Auf dem Weg zu einem prosperierenden europäischen eHealth-Markt–Hindernisse ohne Ausweg, *Telemedizinführer Deutschland*, pp. 292-296, Available Online: http://www.xn--telemedizinfhrer-uzb.de/free/2008/reiher_292_296.pdf [Accessed: October 25, 2021]

Rifi, N., Rachkidi, E., Agoulmine, N., & Taher, N. C. (2017). Towards using blockchain technology for eHealth data access management, *Fourth International Conference on Advances in Biomedical Engineering (ICABME)*, pp. 1-4, Available Online: https://ieeexplore.ieee.org/abstract/document/8167555 [Accessed: October 22, 2021]

Rinsche, F. (2017). The Role of Digital Health Care Startups, *Crossing Borders - Innovation in the U.S. Health Care System: Schriften zur Gesundheitsökonomie*, vol. 84, pp. 185-195, Available Online: https://epub.uni-bayreuth.de/3456 [Accessed: October 24, 2021]

Sanyal, C., Stolee, P., Juzwishin, D., & Husereau, D. (2018). Economic evaluations of eHealth technologies: A systematic review, *PLOS ONE*, vol. 13, no. 6, Available Online: https://doi.org/10.1371/journal.pone.0198112 [Accessed: October 24, 2021]

Schaltegger, S., & Wagner, M. (2011). Sustainable entrepreneurship and sustainability innovation: categories and interactions, *Business strategy and the environment*, vol. 20, no. 4, pp. 222-237, Available Online: https://onlinelibrary.wiley.com/doi/full/10.1002/bse.682 [Accessed: October 24, 2021]

Schweitzer, J., & Synowiec, C. (2012). The Economics of eHealth and mHealth, *Journal of Health Communication*, vol. 17, pp. 73-81, Available Online: https://doi.org/10.1080/10810730.2011.649158 [Accessed: October 21, 2021]

Shaw, T., McGregor, D., Brunner, M., Keep, M., Janssen, A., & Barnet, S. (2017). What is eHealth (6)? Development of a Conceptual Model for eHealth: Qualitative Study with Key Informants, *J Med Internet Res*, vol. 19, no. 10, pp. 1-8, Available Online: https://www.jmir.org/2017/10/e324 [Accessed: October 20, 2021]

Sousa, V., & Dunn Lopez, K. (2017). Towards Usable E-Health. A Systematic Review of Usability Questionnaires, *Applied clinical informatics*, vol. 8, no. 2, pp. 470–490. Availabe Online: https://doi.org/10.4338/ACI-2016-10-R-0170 [Accessed: October 21, 2021]

StartUp Health. (2021). Total digital health industry funding worldwide from 2010 to 2020 (in billion U.S. dollars), Available Online: https://www-statista-com.ludwig.lub.lu.se/statistics/388858/investor-funding-in-digital-health-industry/ [Accessed: October 20, 2021]

Stroetmann, K., Jones, T., Dobrev, A., & Stroetmann, V. (2006). eHealth is Worth it: The economic benefits of implemented eHealth solutions at ten European sites, European Communities, pp. 21-24, Available Online: https://leadership2017.eu/fileadmin/ehealth_impact/documents/ehealthimpactsept2006.pdf [Accessed: October 21, 2021]

Thompson, M. (2021). Digital health is a vital tool: here's how we can make it more sustainable, Available Online: https://theconversation.com/digital-health-is-a-vital-tool-heres-how-we-can-make-it-more-sustainable-165633 [Accessed: October 23, 2021]

United Nations. (2017). Resolution 71/313: Work of the Statistical Commission pertaining to the 2030 Agenda for Sustainable Development, pp. 1-18, Available Online: https://undocs.org/A/RES/71/313 [Accessed: October 23, 2021]

Van Gemert-Pijnen, L., Kelders, S.M., Kip, H., & Sanderman, R. (2018). eHealth Research, Theory and Development: A Multidisciplinary Approach, p. 50, Available Online: https://doi.org/10.4324/9781315385907 [Accessed: October 21, 2021]

Viswanath, K., & Kreuter, M. W. (2007). Health Disparities, Communication Inequalities, and eHealth, *American Journal of Preventive Medicine*, vol. 32, no. 5, pp. 131-133, Available Online: https://www.sciencedirect.com/science/article/pii/S0749379707001006 [Accessed: October 23, 2021]

Wade, V.A., Karnon, J., Elshaug, A.G., & Hiller, J.E. (2010). A systematic review of economic analyses of telehealth services using real time video communication, *BMC Health Serv Res*, vol. 10, no. 233, p. 7. Available Online: https://doi.org/10.1186/1472-6963-10-233 [Accessed: October 21, 2021]

World Commission on Environment and Development. (1987). Our Common Future, p. 27, Available Online: https://sustainabledevelopment.un.org/content/documents/5987our-common-future.pdf [Accessed: October 23, 2021]

Yellowlees, P.M., Chorba, K., Burke Parish, M., Wynn-Jones, H., & Nafiz, N. (2010). Telemedicine can make healthcare greener, *Telemedicine and e-Health*, vol. 16, no. 2, pp. 229-232, Available Online: https://www.liebertpub.com/doi/10.1089/tmj.2009.0105 [Accessed: October 24, 2021]

# YOUR KNOWLEDGE HAS VALUE

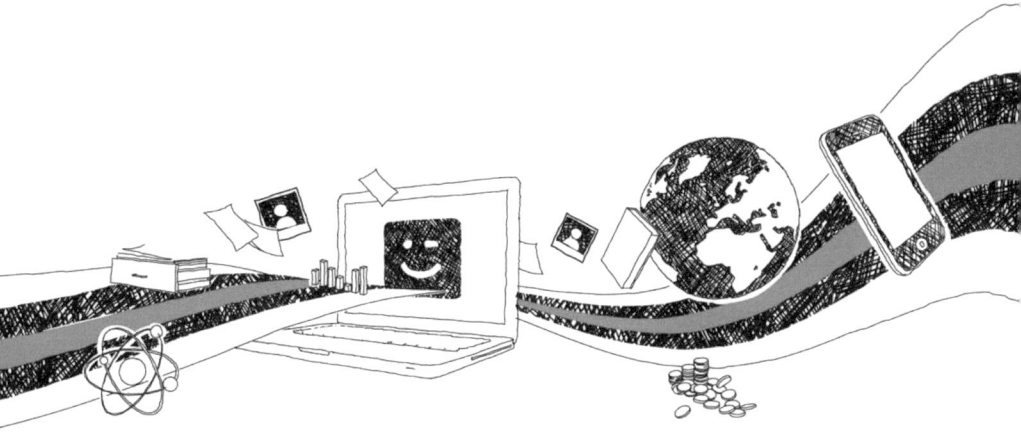

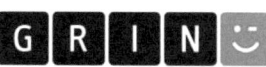